The Longevity Equation:

Unlocking The Secrets To A Longer, Healthier Life

Written by

Dr. Calvin Zeus

asserts the author's ownership of this Book and specifies that no part of the book may be reproduced without permission from the publisher.

Table Of Contents

The Extended View: Transitioning from Rapid Mortality to Gradual Decline

Imagine standing at the edge of a river, watching the relentless current sweep away everything in its path. That's how fast death feels. It's abrupt, sudden, like a thief in the night. But there's another kind of death, one that creeps up slowly, like the tide inching its way up the shore. This is slow death, the gradual decline that many of us will face as we age. Understanding the shift from rapid mortality to this gradual decline is essential for improving how we live our later years. In the past, infectious diseases were the primary cause of death. People died quickly from ailments like tuberculosis, smallpox, or the flu. Advances in medicine, such as antibiotics and vaccines, have dramatically reduced these instances. Today, we face chronic diseases that kill slowly: heart disease, cancer, diabetes, and also neurodegenerative diseases. These aren't sudden, catastrophic events but long, drawn-out battles that can last for decades.

Take heart disease, for example. It doesn't strike out of the blue. It builds up over time, the result of years of poor diet, lack of exercise, and other lifestyle choices. Plaque slowly accumulates in the arteries, restricting blood flow and eventually leading to heart attacks or strokes. But here's the thing – this process takes years, sometimes even decades. By understanding this, we can start to make changes long before the disease reaches its critical point. The same goes for cancer. While some cancers are aggressive and fast-moving, many develop slowly. Colon cancer, for instance, often starts as small polyps in the lining of the intestine. These polyps can take years to turn into malignant tumors. Regular screenings can catch them early, often before they become life-threatening. This is a key point – early detection and prevention can significantly alter the trajectory of these diseases.

Then there's diabetes, particularly type 2 diabetes. It's

a classic example of a slow, progressive condition. The body becomes resistant to insulin over many years, often due to poor dietary habits and lack of physical activity. By the time it's diagnosed, significant damage might already have occurred. But with early intervention, such as dietary changes, exercise, and medication, it's possible to manage the condition and prevent severe complications.

Neurodegenerative diseases like Alzheimer's also exemplify gradual decline. These diseases don't manifest overnight. The brain changes associated with Alzheimer's can start 20 years before symptoms appear. By the time memory loss and cognitive decline are noticeable, substantial damage has already been done. Understanding this long lead time opens up possibilities for early interventions, potentially slowing the disease's progression.

The transition from rapid mortality to gradual decline means that the causes of death are no longer external forces we have little control over but internal processes that we can influence. This shift gives us an incredible opportunity to improve our healthspan – the number of years we live in good health, free from the debilitating effects of chronic disease.

Lifestyle choices play a massive role here. Take smoking, for instance. It's a leading cause of both heart disease and cancer. But quitting smoking, even later in life, can significantly reduce the risk of these diseases. It's a prime example of how lifestyle changes can impact our health trajectory.

Diet is another crucial factor. A diet high in processed foods, sugar, and unhealthy fats contributes to obesity, diabetes, heart disease, and cancer. On the other hand, a diet rich in fruits, vegetables, lean proteins, and healthy fats can reduce the risk of these diseases. It's not just about adding years to our lives but adding life to our years.

Exercise, too, plays a vital role. Regular physical activity helps maintain a healthy weight, reduces blood pressure, improves heart health, and can even lower the risk of certain cancers. It's one of the most powerful tools we have to combat the slow decline of chronic disease. And it's never too late to start. Even moderate exercise, like walking, can have significant benefits, especially for older adults.

Sleep and stress management are also critical. Poor sleep has been linked to a range of health issues, including heart disease, diabetes, and obesity. Chronic stress can exacerbate these conditions, leading to a vicious cycle of declining health. Prioritizing good sleep hygiene and finding effective stress management techniques can make a huge difference.

Prevention and early detection are paramount. Regular check-ups and screenings can catch potential health issues before they become serious problems. Blood pressure checks, cholesterol tests, cancer screenings – these are all tools that can help us stay ahead of the curve. They allow us to take action early, when interventions are most effective.

But it's not just about physical health. Mental and emotional well-being play a crucial role in our overall healthspan. Chronic stress, depression, and anxiety can take a toll on our physical health, exacerbating conditions like heart disease and diabetes. Finding ways to manage stress, stay connected with others, and maintain a positive outlook can improve both our mental and physical health.

Community and support systems are vital. As we age, maintaining strong social connections can help us stay active and engaged, reducing the risk of mental health issues and even physical decline. Whether it's through family, friends, or community groups, staying connected can make a big difference.

In the end, the shift from rapid mortality to gradual decline means that we have more control over our health than ever before. By understanding the long-term nature of chronic diseases and taking proactive steps to prevent and manage them, we can improve our healthspan and enjoy a higher quality of life as we age. It's about making small, sustainable changes that add up over time, helping us live not just longer but better.

Advanced Medicine: Redefining Healthcare for Chronic Illness

Visualize walking into a doctor's office and, instead of treating a symptom with a pill, your physician uses advanced data analysis, genetics, and lifestyle assessments to create a tailored plan for your long-term health. This is the essence of advanced medicine, which shifts the focus from treating acute illnesses to managing chronic diseases in a personalized way. Chronic illnesses like diabetes, heart disease, and cancer aren't just medical issues; they are personal battles that each patient fights differently. Traditional healthcare often treats these diseases in a one-size-fits-all manner, but advanced medicine aims to redefine this approach.

Let's start with genetics. Imagine doctors having access

to your genetic information, allowing them to predict your risk for certain diseases. For instance, BRCA1 and BRCA2 gene mutations are linked to a higher risk of breast and ovarian cancers. With genetic testing, women with these mutations can opt for more frequent screenings or preventive measures, potentially saving lives. This personalized approach means healthcare isn't just reactive; it's proactive.

It anticipates problems and addresses them before they become untreatable and very hard to treat disease or disorder. Consider diabetes management. Traditional treatments focus on managing blood sugar levels with medication and lifestyle changes. Advanced medicine goes further by analyzing each patient's unique response to treatment. Continuous glucose monitors provide real-time data, allowing doctors to tweak treatment plans on the fly. Additionally, researchers are exploring how gut microbiomes affect insulin resistance. By understanding these complex interactions, we can develop more effective, personalized treatments for diabetes.

Heart disease, the leading cause of death worldwide, has also seen advancements. Coronary artery disease, for instance, can now be managed with the help of wearable technology. Devices like smartwatches monitor heart rate and detect irregularities, alerting users and doctors to potential issues before they escalate. Moreover, artificial intelligence (AI) algorithms analyze data from these devices, identifying patterns and providing insights that were previously impossible to detect. This kind of continuous monitoring and data analysis transforms heart disease management from episodic check-ups to constant vigilance.

Cancer treatment is perhaps where advanced medicine shows its most dramatic impact. Traditional chemotherapy attacks cancer cells but also harms healthy cells, causing severe side effects. Enter immunotherapy, which trains the patient's immune system to target cancer cells specifically.

Treatments like CAR-T cell therapy, where a patient's T cells are modified to attack cancer, have shown promising results, particularly in blood cancers. Precision medicine takes it a step further by tailoring treatments based on the genetic profile of both the patient and the tumor. This means that two patients with the same type of cancer might receive entirely different treatments based on their genetic makeup.

Lifestyle and environment also play a significant role in the management of chronic diseases. Advanced medicine doesn't just consider what medications you're taking but also how you live your life. For instance, wearable fitness trackers provide data on physical activity, sleep patterns, and even stress levels. This information helps doctors understand how lifestyle factors contribute to a patient's overall health. By integrating this data into treatment plans, physicians can offer more holistic and effective care.

Artificial intelligence and machine learning are revolutionizing how we approach healthcare. These technologies analyze vast amounts of data, from medical records to genetic information, identifying patterns that human doctors might miss. For example, AI algorithms can predict which patients are at higher risk of complications after surgery, allowing for preventive measures. They can also help in diagnosing diseases earlier and more accurately. Radiologists use AI to analyze medical images, detecting abnormalities with a level of precision that enhances human expertise.

Telemedicine has also emerged as a game-changer, especially during the COVID-19 pandemic. Patients with chronic illnesses often need regular monitoring and consultations. Telemedicine allows them to receive care without leaving their homes, reducing the risk of exposure to infections. Remote monitoring devices can transmit vital signs to healthcare providers in real time, ensuring that patients receive timely interventions. This kind of accessibility is crucial for managing chronic diseases, where consistent monitoring and quick responses can prevent complications.

Personalized nutrition is another frontier in advanced medicine. Diet plays a crucial role in managing chronic diseases, but what works for one person might not work for another. Nutrigenomics studies how genes affect a person's response to nutrients. By analyzing genetic data, doctors can provide dietary recommendations tailored to an individual's genetic makeup. This personalized approach can help manage conditions like obesity, diabetes, and cardiovascular diseases more effectively than generic dietary advice. The integration of mental health into chronic disease management is also gaining attention. Chronic illnesses often take a toll on mental health, and untreated mental health issues can exacerbate physical conditions. Advanced medicine recognizes this interplay and advocates for a more integrated approach. For instance, patients with chronic pain might benefit from therapies that address both the physical and psychological aspects of pain. Cognitive-behavioral therapy, mindfulness, and stress management techniques are becoming part of comprehensive treatment plans.

Moreover, the role of big data in healthcare cannot be overstated. The vast amounts of data generated by electronic health records, wearable devices, and genetic testing provide a treasure trove of information. Analyzing this data can reveal trends and insights that lead to better treatment strategies. For example, big data analytics can help identify which populations are at higher risk for certain diseases, leading to targeted public health interventions. It can also improve the efficiency of healthcare systems by predicting patient admissions and optimizing resource allocation.

The shift to advanced medicine also involves empowering patients. With access to their health data and the tools to understand it, patients can take a more active role in their care. Health apps and online portals allow patients to track their progress, communicate with healthcare providers, and make informed decisions about their treatment. This level of engagement can lead to better adherence to treatment plans and improved health outcomes. Regenerative medicine is another exciting area. Techniques like stem cell therapy hold the promise of repairing damaged tissues and organs. For example, researchers are exploring how to use stem cells to regenerate heart tissue after a heart attack or to treat degenerative diseases like osteoarthritis. While still in the experimental stages, these therapies offer hope for conditions that currently have no cure.

Lastly, advanced medicine emphasizes the importance of continuous learning and adaptation. The medical field is constantly evolving, with new research and technologies emerging at a rapid pace. Healthcare providers must stay updated on the latest advancements and be willing to adapt their practices accordingly. This dynamic approach ensures that patients receive the most current and effective treatments available.

In essence, advanced medicine is about taking a proactive, personalized, and data-driven approach to healthcare. It's about using the latest technologies and research to anticipate health issues before they become severe, tailoring treatments to individual needs, and integrating all aspects of a person's life into their care plan. This shift promises not only to extend our lives but to enhance the quality of those years, turning the fight against chronic disease into a more manageable, and often winnable, battle.

Plan, Strategy, Actions

Every journey needs a map, especially when it involves navigating the complex world of health and longevity. Think of it as a detailed plan, broken down into strategy and actionable steps, to transform your approach to well-being.

We start with the plan. Picture your health as a long-term project, something that needs consistent attention and thoughtful planning. The goal isn't just to live longer but to live better. This means maintaining vitality, staying active, and preventing diseases before they start. The plan section of this book lays out the blueprint. It helps you understand your current health status, identify risk factors, and set realistic, achievable goals. It's like having a roadmap that points you in the right direction.

Next, we move to strategy. Strategy is where the planning turns into a game plan. Imagine you're a coach designing a playbook for your team. You need to consider all the variables: the strengths and weaknesses of your players, the conditions of the playing field, and the tactics of your opponents. In the context of health, this means looking at your lifestyle, diet, exercise routine, and even your mental health. It's about understanding how all these elements interact and influence each other. For example, if you're trying to lower your risk of heart disease, your strategy might include a combination of dietary changes, regular physical activity, and stress management techniques. Each component of your strategy should be evidence-based, drawing on the latest scientific research.

Finally, we get to actions. This is where the rubber meets the road. Actions are the specific steps you take daily to execute your strategy. It's not enough to know that exercise is good for you; you need to incorporate it into your routine. The actions section of this book provides practical advice and step-by-step guides. Think of it as turning strategy into habits. For example, if part of your strategy is to improve your diet, the actions might include meal planning, cooking healthy recipes, and learning to read nutrition labels. It's about making small, sustainable changes that add up over time.

Consider sleep, for instance. We know that good sleep is vital for health, but many of us struggle to get enough quality rest. The plan might start by assessing your current sleep habits and identifying obstacles.

The strategy could involve creating a bedtime routine, limiting screen time before bed, and making your bedroom conducive to sleep. The actions would be the specific steps: setting a consistent bedtime, using blackout curtains, and practicing relaxation techniques.

Or take exercise. The plan could begin with a fitness assessment, understanding your current level of activity and identifying areas for improvement. The strategy might involve setting specific fitness goals, choosing activities you enjoy, and finding ways to stay motivated. The actions are the workouts themselves: scheduling regular exercise sessions, tracking your progress, and adjusting your routine as needed.

Diet is another crucial area. Your plan might involve

evaluating your current eating habits, identifying unhealthy patterns, and setting nutritional goals. The strategy could include learning about balanced diets, incorporating more whole foods, and reducing processed foods and sugar. The actions would be the daily choices: preparing healthy meals, choosing nutritious snacks, and staying hydrated.

Mental health is just as important as physical health. Your plan could start with a mental health check-up, understanding your stress levels, and identifying triggers. The strategy might involve developing coping mechanisms, finding time for relaxation, and seeking professional help if needed. The actions could include practicing mindfulness, scheduling downtime, and connecting with loved ones.

This book also emphasizes the importance of regular check-ups and screenings. The plan might involve scheduling routine visits with your healthcare provider, understanding which screenings you need based on your age and risk factors, and staying on top of vaccinations. The strategy could include maintaining an organized health record, staying informed about new screening guidelines, and advocating for yourself in medical settings. The actions are the appointments themselves: making and keeping doctor's appointments, following through with recommended tests, and discussing any concerns with your healthcare provider.

Implementing these steps requires commitment and consistency. It's not about making drastic changes overnight but about integrating small, manageable steps into your daily life. For example, if you want to reduce your sugar intake, you might start by cutting out sugary drinks, then gradually reduce added sugars in your meals, and finally, learn to satisfy your sweet tooth with healthier alternatives like fruits.

Motivation can wane, and life can get in the way, but that's where the action steps help. They break down your strategy into bite-sized tasks that feel achievable. For example, if your goal is to exercise more, an action step could be setting a goal to walk 10,000 steps a day. Use a pedometer or smartphone app to track your progress. Each step you take is a small victory that brings you closer to your overall goal.

Another key aspect is tracking your progress. This book guides you on how to monitor your health journey, from keeping a food diary to tracking your fitness achievements. It's about celebrating the small wins and learning from setbacks. For instance, if you aim to lower your blood pressure, regular monitoring helps you see how your lifestyle changes impact your readings.

Remember, this journey is personal. What works for one person might not work for another. This book encourages you to customize your plan, strategy, and actions based on your unique needs and circumstances. For example, if you're managing a chronic condition like diabetes, your plan might include regular blood sugar monitoring, your strategy might involve specific dietary adjustments, and your actions could include preparing balanced meals and staying active.

Support systems play a significant role too. This book advises on building a network of support, whether it's family, friends, or a healthcare team. They can provide encouragement, hold you accountable, and offer help when needed. For instance, if you're trying to quit smoking, having a support group or a buddy can make a huge difference.

Life is unpredictable, and sometimes plans need to change. It's okay to adjust your strategy and actions as needed. For example, if you're traveling and can't stick to your usual exercise routine, find ways to stay active on the go, like taking the stairs instead of the elevator or doing bodyweight exercises in your hotel room.

In essence, taking control of your health in a structured yet flexible way is about understanding where you are now, where you want to be, and how to get there. It's a journey of continuous improvement, learning, and adaptation, ensuring that you not only add years to your life but also life to

your years.

Longevity Champions: Health Improvements with Age

Imagine you're watching a marathon. As the runners reach the halfway point, many start to slow down, some drop out, but a few seem to find their stride, gaining momentum as they push forward. These are the longevity champions – people who improve their health and vitality as they age. They don't just endure the marathon of life;

they thrive, setting a pace that defies the typical narrative of aging.

Take the story of Fauja Singh, who ran his first marathon at age 89 and continued to run well into his 100s. What sets people like Singh apart isn't just luck or genetics; it's a combination of lifestyle choices, mindset, and sometimes, a bit of serendipity. These longevity champions show us that it's possible to maintain and even enhance health as the years go by.

One key to this remarkable endurance is physical activity. Regular exercise isn't just about keeping fit; it's about maintaining and improving bodily functions. Studies have shown that physical activity can delay the onset of chronic diseases, boost mental health, and improve overall quality of life. For instance, a study published in the *British Journal of Sports Medicine* found that older adults who engage in regular physical activity have a lower risk of heart disease, stroke, and certain types of cancer. Exercise helps maintain muscle mass, improve balance, and enhance cognitive function, which are all crucial as we age.

Diet plays another significant role in the health of longevity champions. Consider the Mediterranean diet, rich in fruits, vegetables, whole grains, olive oil, and lean protein. Research from the *New England Journal of Medicine* indicates that this diet can reduce the risk of heart disease, improve brain health, and even extend lifespan. It's not about strict diets or extreme measures; it's about making sustainable, healthy choices that become a natural part of life.

Sleep is often overlooked but is critical to health. Quality sleep helps repair the body, consolidate memory, and regulate mood. Studies suggest that older adults who maintain good sleep habits have better physical and mental health. For example, research in the "**Journal of Clinical Sleep Medicine**" shows that adults who get seven to eight hours of sleep per night have lower rates of heart disease and depression. Simple changes, like maintaining a consistent sleep schedule, creating a restful environment, and avoiding screens before bed, can make a significant difference.

Social connections are another vital component. Loneliness and social isolation can lead to a host of health problems, including depression and cardiovascular disease. On the flip side, strong social ties can improve mental health, boost the immune system, and even increase longevity. The *Journal of Health and Social Behavior* published findings that older adults with robust social networks live longer and enjoy better health. Regular social interaction provides emotional support, reduces stress, and gives a sense of purpose.

Mental attitude also matters. The mind-body connection is powerful, and a positive outlook can have tangible health benefits. Studies have shown that optimism and a sense of purpose are linked to lower risks of chronic diseases and longer life. For instance, research in the *American Journal of Epidemiology* found that individuals with a positive attitude towards aging live longer and have a lower risk of major illnesses. Cultivating a positive mindset can involve mindfulness practices, staying engaged in hobbies, and setting new goals. Consider the Blue Zones, areas around the world where people live significantly longer lives. Places like Okinawa in Japan, Sardinia in Italy, and Loma Linda in California are home to some of the world's longest-living people. What do they have in common? A combination of healthy diet, regular physical activity, strong social ties, and a sense of purpose. They move naturally throughout the day, eat plant-based diets, engage in social activities, and have a positive outlook on life. These communities provide real-world examples of how lifestyle choices can impact longevity.

Even when faced with health challenges, many longevity champions adapt and find ways to thrive. Consider the story of Diana Nyad, who at age 64 became the first person to swim from Cuba to Florida without a shark cage. Her achievement wasn't just about physical endurance but also mental resilience. Nyad's story highlights the importance of perseverance and adaptability in the face of obstacles. Whether dealing with chronic conditions or recovering from illness, the ability to adapt and stay active is crucial for maintaining health.

Technology also plays a role in supporting longevity. Wearable devices can track physical activity, sleep patterns, and even detect irregular heartbeats. Telemedicine allows for regular check-ups without leaving home, making healthcare more accessible. These tools empower individuals to take charge of their health, providing real-time feedback and facilitating early detection of potential issues.

Mental stimulation is another key factor. Keeping the brain active through learning, puzzles, reading, or social interaction helps maintain cognitive function. The *Journal of the American Medical Association* published research showing that engaging in mentally stimulating activities can delay the onset of dementia and improve cognitive health. Lifelong learning and curiosity can keep the mind sharp and engaged.

Maintaining a sense of purpose can't be overstated. Whether through work, volunteering, or pursuing hobbies, having a reason to get up in the morning provides motivation and fulfillment. Purpose-driven individuals tend to live longer and healthier lives, as shown in a study by the *Journal of Psychological Science*, which found a strong link between purpose in life and longevity.

Emotional health is equally important. Managing stress through techniques like meditation, yoga, and deep-breathing exercises can improve overall health. Chronic stress has been linked to numerous health problems, including heart disease and weakened immune function. Learning to manage stress effectively is a cornerstone of longevity.

In essence, becoming a longevity champion involves a multifaceted approach to health. It's about integrating physical activity, a balanced diet, quality sleep, social connections, mental stimulation, and a positive attitude into daily life. It's about making choices that support long-term health and well-being, adapting to challenges, and maintaining a sense of purpose and joy. These champions show us that it's possible to not only extend our lives but to enhance the quality of those extra years, turning the journey of aging into a path of continued growth and vitality.

Caloric Restriction and Longevity: Insights into Hunger and Wellness

Employing a diet where eating less doesn't mean starving but rather living longer and healthier. This is the concept behind caloric restriction, a practice that has gained significant attention for its potential to extend lifespan and improve wellness. By reducing caloric intake without malnutrition, scientists believe we can unlock some of the secrets to longevity.

At its core, caloric restriction involves consuming fewer calories than usual while ensuring that all necessary nutrients are included in the diet. The idea isn't to drastically cut food but to create a balanced, nutrient-dense diet that supports health while slightly reducing energy intake. Studies in various organisms, from yeast to monkeys, have shown that caloric restriction can extend lifespan and delay the onset of age-related diseases. For instance, research on rodents has consistently demonstrated that those on a restricted diet live up to 40% longer than their well-fed counterparts.

How does this work? One theory suggests that caloric restriction reduces metabolic rate and oxidative stress, which are linked to the aging process. When we eat, our bodies convert food into energy, producing free radicals as a byproduct. These free radicals can damage cells over time, contributing to aging and disease. By eating less, we generate fewer free radicals, potentially slowing down this damage. A study published in *Nature Communications* supports this, showing that caloric restriction reduces the production of reactive oxygen species, molecules that can harm cells and accelerate aging.

Another fascinating aspect of caloric restriction is its impact on genetic expression. Research indicates that reducing calorie intake can activate certain genes associated with longevity. For example, caloric restriction has been shown to upregulate the SIRT1 gene, often called the "longevity gene." This gene is involved in cellular repair and maintenance, processes crucial for healthy aging. A study in *Cell Reports* highlights that SIRT1 activation can improve metabolic efficiency and increase stress resistance, both important factors for a longer, healthier life.

Human studies on caloric restriction are more challenging due to ethical and practical considerations, but the evidence is promising. The CALERIE (Comprehensive Assessment of Long-term Effects of Reducing Intake of Energy) trial, funded by the National Institute on Aging, is one of the most significant studies in this area. Over two years, participants reduced their caloric intake by 25%. The results showed improvements in markers of cardiovascular health, insulin sensitivity, and inflammation, all of which are linked to longevity.

Beyond the biological mechanisms, caloric restriction may also affect hunger and satiety hormones, potentially altering our relationship with food. Ghrelin, known as the "hunger hormone," increases appetite, while leptin, the "satiety hormone," signals fullness. Studies have found that caloric restriction can stabilize these hormones, reducing constant hunger and making it easier to maintain a balanced diet. Research published in *Endocrinology* found that caloric restriction increased ghrelin sensitivity, meaning that the body becomes more efficient at regulating hunger signals, which helps prevent overeating and obesity.

However, it's important to approach caloric restriction cautiously. It requires careful planning to ensure that all nutritional needs are met. This isn't about severe dieting or malnutrition; it's about finding a sustainable way to eat less while still nourishing the body. Consulting with healthcare professionals before making significant dietary changes is crucial to avoid potential health risks.

Intermittent fasting, a related practice, involves alternating periods of eating and fasting. This method also shows promise for promoting longevity and health. Studies suggest that intermittent fasting can improve metabolic health, reduce inflammation, and enhance cellular repair processes. A review in **"The New England Journal of Medicine"** concluded that intermittent fasting can improve biomarkers of disease, reduce oxidative stress, and preserve learning and memory functioning, similar to caloric restriction.

One practical approach to incorporating caloric restriction is to focus on nutrient-dense foods that provide more vitamins and minerals for fewer calories. Vegetables, fruits, whole grains, lean proteins, and healthy fats are essential components of a calorically restricted diet. These foods help ensure that even with fewer calories, the body receives the nutrients it needs to function optimally.

Another strategy is to reduce portion sizes gradually. Rather than making drastic cuts, slowly decreasing the amount of food on your plate can help the body adjust to a lower calorie intake without feeling deprived. This gradual approach also makes it easier to maintain the diet over the long term, which is essential for reaping the potential longevity benefits.

Mindful eating can also support caloric restriction. By paying attention to hunger and fullness cues, eating slowly, and savoring each bite, we can become more in tune with our body's needs. This practice can help prevent overeating and make it easier to adhere to a calorically restricted diet. Research in *Appetite* found that mindful eating techniques can significantly reduce caloric intake while enhancing the enjoyment and satisfaction of meals. It's also worth noting that the effects of caloric restriction may vary depending on individual factors such as genetics, age, and overall health. What works for one person might not work for another, so it's essential to personalize any dietary changes. Continuous monitoring and adjustments, guided by healthcare professionals, can help optimize the benefits while minimizing risks.

Despite the potential benefits, caloric restriction isn't a magic bullet. It should be part of a broader approach to health and wellness that includes regular physical activity, stress management, and social connections. Longevity isn't just about living longer but living well, with vitality and purpose.

In essence, caloric restriction offers a fascinating glimpse into how we might extend our lives and improve our health by simply eating less. It's a reminder that sometimes, less truly can be more, especially when it comes to nourishing our bodies and minds. By understanding and applying the principles of caloric restriction, we can take a proactive step towards a healthier, longer life.

Modern Diet Dilemma: Can Our Ancestral DNA Adapt?

Our ancestors thrived on a diet of wild game, fruits, and roots. Fast forward to today, and our plates are filled with processed foods, sugars, and grains. This stark contrast between past and present diets raises a pressing question: Can our ancestral DNA adapt to our modern diet, or are we setting ourselves up for health issues by straying so far from our evolutionary roots?

Our genetic makeup was shaped over thousands of years when food was scarce, and survival depended on hunting and gathering. The diet of our Paleolithic ancestors was rich in lean proteins, omega-3 fatty acids, fiber, and essential vitamins and minerals, but low in carbohydrates and sugars. Their lifestyle required a lot of physical activity, which complemented their diet. Fast forward to the agricultural revolution about 10,000 years ago, and our diet started to change. We began cultivating grains and domesticating animals, which introduced new foods into our diets. However, our genes haven't fully caught up with these dietary changes. Today, our modern diet is a far cry from the ancestral diet. Highly processed foods, refined sugars, and artificial additives dominate our meals. These foods are convenient but often stripped of nutritional value, leading to overconsumption and health problems. Obesity, diabetes, heart disease, and other chronic conditions have become rampant. The problem is compounded by our sedentary lifestyles, which contrast sharply with the active lives of our ancestors.

Our bodies are still wired to expect the nutrient-rich, unprocessed foods our ancestors ate. For instance, our taste buds are designed to favor sweet, salty, and fatty foods because they were rare and valuable energy sources in the past. In today's world, these foods are abundant, and our instinctual cravings can lead to overeating and weight gain. Our genes haven't adapted to the constant availability of high-calorie foods, leading to a mismatch between our biology and our environment. One major issue is the rapid increase in carbohydrate consumption. Ancient diets were low in refined carbohydrates, while modern diets are often high in sugar and refined grains. This shift has had significant impacts on our health. Refined carbohydrates cause rapid spikes in blood sugar, leading to insulin resistance and type 2 diabetes.

Research published in the "**Journal of Clinical Endocrinology & Metabolism**" indicates that high carbohydrate intake, especially refined sugars, is linked to an increased risk of metabolic syndrome, a cluster of conditions that increase the risk of heart disease and diabetes.

The role of fats in our diet has also changed dramatically. Our ancestors consumed healthy fats from sources like fish, nuts, and seeds, which are rich in omega-3 fatty acids. Modern diets, however, are high in unhealthy trans fats and omega-6 fatty acids found in processed and fried foods. An imbalance between omega-3 and omega-6 fatty acids can lead to chronic inflammation, a key factor in many chronic diseases. A study in "**Prostaglandins, Leukotrienes, and Essential**

Fatty Acids" suggests that a higher ratio of omega-6 to omega-3 fatty acids is associated with increased inflammation and a higher risk of chronic diseases.

Protein intake has also shifted. While our ancestors relied on wild game and plant-based proteins, modern diets often include large amounts of red and processed meats. These types of meat have been linked to higher risks of heart disease, cancer, and other health issues. In contrast, plant-based proteins and lean meats, such as fish and poultry, offer a healthier alternative. Research in the **"Journal of the American Medical Association"** shows that replacing red and processed meats with plant-based proteins can lower the risk of mortality and chronic diseases.

Another significant difference is the fiber content in our diets. Our ancestors consumed large amounts of fiber from fruits, vegetables, nuts, and seeds. Fiber is essential for digestive health, helps regulate blood sugar levels, and reduces the risk of cardiovascular diseases. Modern diets, however, are often low in fiber due to the high consumption of processed foods. The lack of fiber can lead to digestive problems, weight gain, and increased risk of chronic diseases. The **"American Journal of Clinical Nutrition"** published findings that high dietary fiber intake is associated with a reduced risk of developing cardiovascular disease and type 2 diabetes.

Additionally, the variety and diversity of foods have decreased. Our ancestors ate a wide range of plants and animals, providing a diverse array of nutrients. Modern diets tend to rely on a smaller selection of foods, leading to nutritional deficiencies. For example, many people don't get enough vitamins and minerals essential for health, such as vitamin D, magnesium, and potassium. This lack of diversity can contribute to health issues and affect overall well-being. Research in "**Nature**" shows that dietary diversity is crucial for maintaining a healthy gut microbiome, which plays a vital role in immune function, digestion, and overall health.

The question remains: Can our DNA adapt to these rapid changes in our diet? Evolutionary changes take thousands of years, so it's unlikely that our genes will catch up with our modern diet anytime soon. Instead, the focus should be on adapting our diets to better match our genetic makeup. This means prioritizing whole, unprocessed foods, reducing refined carbohydrates and sugars, increasing healthy fats and proteins, and ensuring adequate fiber intake. Adopting dietary patterns similar to those of our ancestors, such as the Paleo or Mediterranean diets, can help bridge the gap between our current diets and what our bodies are designed to handle. These diets emphasize whole foods, lean proteins, healthy fats, and plenty of fruits and vegetables. By aligning our diets more closely with our genetic expectations, we can improve our health and reduce the risk of chronic diseases.

Incorporating these dietary changes doesn't mean abandoning modern conveniences entirely. It's about making informed choices and finding a balance that works for our individual needs. Simple changes, like choosing whole grains over refined grains, snacking on nuts and seeds instead of processed snacks, and incorporating more fruits and vegetables into meals, can make a significant difference. Education and awareness are also critical. Understanding the impact of our dietary choices on our health can empower us to make better decisions. Public health initiatives and nutrition education programs can play a significant role in helping people understand the importance of a balanced, nutrient-dense diet.

Ultimately, while our DNA might not adapt quickly to our modern diet, we can take steps to adapt our eating habits to better align with our evolutionary heritage. By doing so, we can improve our health, increase our vitality, and enhance our quality of life.

Cardiac Focus: Addressing and Preventing the Leading Cause of Death

Heart disease doesn't announce itself with fanfare. It's silent, stealthy, and deadly. We often don't see it coming until it's too late. The heart, a powerful organ pumping life through our veins, can suddenly become vulnerable, weakened by the choices we make daily. This vulnerability is why heart disease remains the leading cause of death worldwide. But while the statistics are daunting, the path to prevention and control is within reach.

Focusing on the Western diet: high in processed foods, loaded with saturated fats, refined sugars, and salt. This diet doesn't just satisfy hunger; it slowly chips away at the health of our arteries, raising blood pressure and cholesterol levels. Plaque begins to build up, a sticky blend of fat, cholesterol, and other substances, narrowing the arteries and reducing blood flow to the heart. This condition, known as atherosclerosis, is the breeding ground for heart attacks, strokes, and other cardiovascular diseases. High blood pressure, often called hypertension, is another major contributor to heart disease. It's like having a fire hose for arteries instead of a garden hose. The increased force of blood against the artery walls damages them over time, making it easier for plaque to form. This is why managing blood pressure is crucial in preventing heart disease. The American Heart Association recommends regular monitoring of blood pressure, aiming to keep it below 120/80 mm Hg.

But diet and blood pressure are just the beginning. Smoking, a habit often started in youth, wreaks havoc on the heart. The chemicals in tobacco damage the lining of the arteries, leading to plaque buildup. Nicotine raises blood pressure, and carbon monoxide reduces the amount of oxygen that the blood can carry. Smoking doesn't just double the risk of heart disease—it quadruples it. Quitting smoking, regardless of age, significantly reduces the risk of heart disease, and the benefits begin almost immediately after stopping.

Physical inactivity is another major factor. Our ancestors were hunters and gatherers, constantly moving, but modern life has become sedentary. We spend hours sitting at desks, in cars, and on couches. This lack of physical activity contributes to obesity, diabetes, and high blood pressure, all of which are major risk factors for heart disease. The Centers for Disease Control and Prevention (CDC) recommends at least 150 minutes of moderate-intensity exercise per week, which can be as simple as brisk walking, to help maintain heart health.

Obesity itself is a significant risk factor. Carrying excess weight strains the heart, raises blood pressure, and increases cholesterol levels. It also raises the risk of developing type 2 diabetes, which further compounds the risk of heart disease. But losing even a small amount of weight can make a big difference. According to the CDC, losing just 5-10% of body weight can lower blood pressure, cholesterol, and blood sugar levels, all of which are beneficial for heart health. Diabetes, particularly type 2, is closely linked to heart disease. High blood sugar from diabetes can damage blood vessels and the nerves that control the heart. Over time, this damage increases the risk of heart disease. In fact, adults with diabetes are nearly twice as likely to die from heart disease or stroke as those without diabetes. Managing blood sugar levels through diet, exercise, and medication is essential in reducing this risk. Stress, often overlooked, is another player in the heart disease game. Chronic stress leads to behaviors and factors that increase heart disease risk: overeating, physical inactivity, smoking, and excessive alcohol use. It can also raise blood pressure and lead to artery damage. Finding ways to manage stress—whether through exercise, meditation, or therapy—is crucial for heart health.

Alcohol consumption is a double-edged sword. While

moderate alcohol consumption has been shown to have some heart benefits, excessive drinking can lead to high blood pressure, heart failure, and even stroke. The key is moderation. The American Heart Association defines moderate drinking as no more than one drink per day for women and two drinks per day for men. Anything beyond this increases the risk of heart disease.

So, what can be done to reduce these risks? A heart-healthy diet is a good place to start. The Mediterranean diet, rich in fruits, vegetables, whole grains, fish, and olive oil, has been shown to reduce the risk of heart disease. This diet is low in red meat, sugar, and saturated fats, all of which contribute to heart disease. Instead, it focuses on foods that are high in fiber, antioxidants, and healthy fats, which help to protect the heart.

Regular physical activity is also crucial. Exercise helps to control weight, lower blood pressure, reduce cholesterol levels, and improve overall cardiovascular health. It doesn't have to be strenuous—a brisk walk, cycling, or swimming can all make a significant difference. The goal is to keep the heart pumping and the blood flowing.

Managing stress is equally important. Chronic stress can contribute to heart disease, so finding ways to relax and decompress is essential. This might include practicing mindfulness, spending time with loved ones, or engaging in hobbies. Reducing stress can lower blood pressure, improve mental health, and reduce the risk of heart disease.

Quitting smoking is perhaps the single most effective thing one can do to protect the heart. The benefits of quitting smoking begin almost immediately, with the risk of heart disease halved after just one year of quitting. It's never too late to quit, and the health benefits are substantial.

Regular health screenings are also essential. Monitoring blood pressure, cholesterol levels, and blood sugar can help catch problems early before they lead to heart disease. Early detection and treatment of these conditions can prevent heart disease and improve overall health. Education and awareness are crucial in the fight against heart disease. Understanding the risk factors and taking steps to reduce them can save lives. Public health initiatives and educational programs can help raise awareness and encourage people to take proactive steps to protect their heart health.

In the end, the power to prevent heart disease is largely in our hands. By making healthy lifestyle choices, managing stress, and staying informed, we can reduce our risk and live longer, healthier lives. It's not about making drastic changes overnight but about making small, sustainable changes that add up to a big difference. The heart is a resilient organ, but it needs our help to stay strong and healthy.

Cancer Control: Innovative Approaches to Combat Cancer

Cancer, a formidable adversary, has plagued humanity for centuries, claiming countless lives. But as our understanding of biology and technology advances, so do the methods we use to combat this disease. Traditional treatments like chemotherapy and radiation have saved many lives, but they often come with severe side effects. Today, innovative approaches are transforming how we diagnose, treat, and even prevent cancer.

One very groundbreaking development is immunotherapy. Unlike traditional treatments that directly target cancer cells, immunotherapy harnesses the body's immune system to fight the disease. The idea is to boost or restore the immune system's ability to identify and destroy cancer cells. One promising type of immunotherapy is checkpoint inhibitors. These drugs work by blocking proteins that prevent the immune system from attacking cancer cells. For instance, drugs like pembrolizumab (Keytruda) and nivolumab (Opdivo) have shown remarkable success in treating advanced melanoma and lung cancer. By unleashing the immune system, these treatments have extended the lives of patients who had few options left.

Another exciting area is CAR T-cell therapy. This approach involves modifying a patient's T cells (a type of immune cell) to recognize and attack cancer cells. The modified T cells are infused back into the patient's body, where they seek out and destroy cancer cells. CAR T-cell therapy has shown extraordinary success in treating certain types of blood cancers, such as acute lymphoblastic leukemia (ALL) and non-Hodgkin lymphoma. In some cases, patients who had exhausted all other treatments have achieved complete remission.

Precision medicine is also revolutionizing cancer treatment. Instead of a one-size-fits-all approach, precision medicine tailors treatment to the individual characteristics of each patient's cancer. By analyzing genetic mutations and other molecular changes in cancer cells, doctors can select therapies that are most likely to be effective. For example, targeted therapies like trastuzumab (Herceptin) for HER2-positive breast cancer and vemurafenib (Zelboraf) for BRAF-mutated melanoma have significantly improved outcomes for patients with these specific mutations.

The CRISPR-Cas9 gene-editing technology is another innovative tool making waves in cancer research. This powerful technology allows scientists to precisely edit genes within cells, opening up new possibilities for cancer treatment. Researchers are exploring ways to use CRISPR to correct genetic mutations that drive cancer growth or to engineer immune cells to better recognize and attack cancer. While still in the early stages, CRISPR holds immense potential for creating highly personalized and effective cancer therapies.

Liquid biopsies represent another major advancement in cancer diagnosis and monitoring. Traditional biopsies require invasive procedures to obtain tissue samples from tumors. Liquid biopsies, on the other hand, use a simple blood draw to detect cancer DNA circulating in the bloodstream. This minimally invasive approach allows for earlier detection of cancer, monitoring of treatment response, and detection of relapse. Liquid biopsies are particularly valuable for cancers that are difficult to biopsy traditionally, such as lung cancer.

Artificial intelligence (AI) and machine learning are also playing an increasingly important role in cancer care. AI algorithms can analyze vast amounts of data to identify patterns and make predictions that can aid in diagnosis and treatment planning. For example, AI can help radiologists detect cancerous lesions in medical images with greater accuracy. Additionally, AI-driven tools can analyze genetic data to identify potential therapeutic targets and predict how patients will respond to specific treatments.

Nanotechnology offers another innovative approach to cancer treatment. Nanoparticles can be designed to deliver drugs directly to cancer cells, minimizing damage to healthy tissue and reducing side effects. These tiny particles can also be engineered to release their payload in response to specific triggers, such as changes in pH or temperature, ensuring that the drugs are activated only in the vicinity of the tumor. Researchers are also exploring the use of nanoparticles for imaging and early detection of cancer.

On the prevention front, vaccines are making strides in reducing the incidence of certain cancers. The human papillomavirus (HPV) vaccine, for example, has been highly effective in preventing HPV-related cancers, including cervical, anal, and throat cancers. By preventing infection with high-risk HPV strains, the vaccine reduces the risk of these cancers developing later in life. Additionally, researchers are working on therapeutic cancer vaccines that aim to treat existing cancers by stimulating the immune system to attack cancer cells. The integration of lifestyle interventions with medical treatments is another promising approach. Research has shown that factors such as diet, exercise, and stress management can influence cancer progression and treatment outcomes. For example, a study published in *JAMA Oncology* found that regular physical activity was associated with a lower risk of cancer recurrence and improved survival in patients with high-risk breast cancer. Similarly, dietary interventions, such as reducing sugar intake and increasing consumption of fruits and vegetables, can support overall health and enhance the effectiveness of cancer treatments.

Collaborative efforts are also accelerating progress in cancer research and treatment. Large-scale initiatives like the Cancer Moonshot, launched by the U.S. government, aim to advance cancer research through increased funding, data sharing, and collaboration among researchers, clinicians, and patients. By fostering a collaborative environment, these initiatives are driving innovation and speeding up the development of new therapies.

Despite these advancements, challenges remain. Cancer is a

complex and heterogeneous disease, with each type and even each patient's cancer presenting unique challenges. Continued research and investment are essential to overcome these challenges and develop more effective treatments. Clinical trials play a critical role in this process, providing valuable data on the safety and efficacy of new therapies. Patients participating in clinical trials contribute to the advancement of cancer treatment and may gain access to cutting-edge therapies not yet available to the public.

Education and awareness are also crucial in the fight against cancer. Public health campaigns that promote cancer prevention, early detection, and access to care can save lives. For example, initiatives that encourage regular screenings for breast, colorectal, and prostate cancers can lead to earlier detection and improved outcomes. Additionally, raising awareness about the importance of a healthy lifestyle can help reduce the overall burden of cancer.

The fight against cancer is multifaceted, involving a combination of innovative treatments, advanced technologies, and preventive measures. While significant progress has been made, the journey is far from over. Continued research, collaboration, and education are key to winning the battle against this formidable disease. By embracing innovation and working together, we can transform cancer care and improve the lives of millions worldwide.

Pursuing Cognitive Health: Exploring Alzheimer's and Other Brain Disorders

Alzheimer's disease, a relentless and progressive brain disorder, robs individuals of their memories, cognitive functions, and ultimately, their independence. This insidious condition is the most common cause of dementia, affecting millions of people worldwide. Despite the significant advancements in medical research, Alzheimer's remains a formidable challenge. However, exploring the latest findings and innovative approaches offers hope in the fight against this and other brain disorders.

The brain, a complex organ, consists of billions of neurons that communicate through electrical and chemical signals. In Alzheimer's, these neurons degenerate and die, disrupting communication, metabolism, and repair mechanisms. The hallmark features of Alzheimer's are amyloid plaques and tau tangles. Amyloid plaques are sticky clumps of protein fragments that accumulate between neurons, while tau tangles are twisted fibers of another protein that build up inside neurons. Together, these abnormalities interfere with neuron function and trigger inflammation, further damaging brain cells.

Early diagnosis of Alzheimer's is critical for managing the disease and improving the quality of life for patients and caregivers. Recent advancements in diagnostic techniques have made it possible to detect Alzheimer's earlier than ever before. Brain imaging technologies like positron emission tomography

(PET) scans can identify amyloid plaques and tau tangles in the brain. Additionally, cerebrospinal fluid (CSF) tests can measure levels of amyloid and tau proteins, providing further evidence of Alzheimer's. These diagnostic tools enable doctors to distinguish Alzheimer's from other forms of dementia and tailor treatments accordingly.

One promising area of research is the development of disease-modifying therapies. Traditional treatments for Alzheimer's primarily focus on alleviating symptoms, but disease-modifying therapies aim to slow or halt the progression of the disease. Aducanumab, an antibody that targets amyloid plaques, received FDA approval in 2021, marking a significant milestone. Although its approval has been controversial, aducanumab represents a shift toward targeting the underlying pathology of Alzheimer's. Ongoing research is exploring other potential therapies, including drugs that target tau tangles, inflammation, and other pathways involved in the disease.

Lifestyle interventions also play a crucial role in maintaining cognitive health and potentially reducing the risk of Alzheimer's. Regular physical exercise, a healthy diet, and cognitive stimulation have been shown to benefit brain health. The Mediterranean diet, rich in fruits, vegetables, whole grains, and healthy fats, has been associated with a lower risk of cognitive decline. Additionally, activities that challenge the brain, such as puzzles, reading, and social engagement, can help preserve cognitive function. These lifestyle choices not only promote overall health but also support brain resilience.

Beyond Alzheimer's, other brain disorders, such as Parkinson's disease, Huntington's disease, and multiple sclerosis (MS), also pose significant challenges. Parkinson's disease, characterized by the loss of dopamine-producing neurons, leads to motor symptoms like tremors, rigidity, and bradykinesia (slowness of movement). Although there is no cure for Parkinson's, medications that increase dopamine levels or mimic its effects can help manage symptoms. Deep brain stimulation (DBS), a surgical procedure that involves implanting electrodes in the brain, has also shown promise in reducing motor symptoms and improving the quality of life for patients with advanced Parkinson's.

Huntington's disease, a genetic disorder, causes the progressive breakdown of nerve cells in the brain. This leads to movement disorders, cognitive decline, and psychiatric symptoms. The disease is caused by a mutation in the HTT gene, which leads to the production of an abnormal protein that gradually damages neurons. While there is no cure for Huntington's, research is focusing on gene-silencing therapies that aim to reduce the production of the toxic protein. Early clinical trials have shown encouraging results, offering hope for individuals with this devastating condition.

Multiple sclerosis, an autoimmune disorder, occurs when the immune system mistakenly attacks the protective covering of nerve fibers (myelin) in the central nervous system. This results in communication problems between the brain and the rest of the body. Symptoms of MS vary widely and can include fatigue, difficulty walking, numbness, and cognitive impairment. Disease-modifying therapies can help manage MS by reducing the frequency and severity of relapses. These therapies work by modulating the immune system to prevent it from attacking myelin. In addition to pharmaceutical approaches, non-pharmacological interventions are gaining attention in the management of brain disorders. Cognitive behavioral therapy (CBT) and other forms of psychotherapy can help individuals cope with the emotional and psychological challenges associated with these conditions. For example, CBT has been shown to be effective in managing anxiety and depression in individuals with Alzheimer's and Parkinson's disease. Occupational therapy and physical therapy can also play a crucial role in maintaining function and improving the quality of life for individuals with brain disorders.

Emerging technologies are also transforming the landscape of brain disorder management. Brain-computer interfaces (BCIs), for example, are being developed to help individuals with severe paralysis communicate and interact with their environment. BCIs work by translating brain signals into commands that can control external devices, such as computers or robotic limbs. While still in the experimental stage, BCIs hold great potential for improving the lives of individuals with conditions like amyotrophic lateral sclerosis (ALS) and spinal cord injuries.

Another exciting development is the use of stem cell therapy to treat brain disorders. Stem cells have the unique ability to develop into various types of cells, including neurons. Researchers are exploring ways to use stem cells to replace damaged neurons and restore function in conditions like Parkinson's and MS. Early studies have shown promising results, but more research is needed to determine the safety and efficacy of stem cell therapies in humans.

Public health initiatives and community support are also essential in addressing the challenges posed by brain disorders. Increasing awareness and understanding of these conditions can reduce stigma and promote early diagnosis and intervention. Support groups and community programs can provide valuable resources and emotional support for individuals with brain disorders and their caregivers. These initiatives help create a more inclusive and supportive environment for those affected by these conditions.

In summary, pursuing cognitive health and addressing brain disorders like Alzheimer's, Parkinson's, Huntington's, and MS requires a multifaceted approach. Advances in diagnostic techniques, disease-modifying therapies, lifestyle interventions, and emerging technologies offer hope for better management and improved outcomes. Ongoing research, public health initiatives, and community support are essential in the fight against these debilitating conditions. By working together and embracing innovation, we can make significant strides in preserving cognitive health and enhancing the quality of life for individuals with brain disorders.

Strategic Thinking: Crafting Effective Health Principles

When it comes to health, a strategic approach can make all the difference. Crafting effective health principles requires a blend of evidence-based knowledge, proactive planning, and adaptability to changing circumstances. Effective health principles serve as a roadmap, guiding individuals and communities toward better health outcomes. By focusing on prevention, understanding the role of lifestyle choices, and leveraging technology, we can create robust strategies for a healthier future. One of the fundamental aspects of strategic health thinking is prioritizing prevention. Rather than waiting for diseases to develop and then treating them, a proactive approach focuses on reducing risk factors and enhancing protective factors.

Vaccination programs are a prime example. Vaccines have drastically reduced the incidence of infectious diseases like measles, polio, and influenza. According to the CDC, vaccines have prevented millions of deaths worldwide and continue to be one of the most cost-effective health interventions available.

Regular health screenings and early detection are also critical components of preventive health strategies. Conditions such as hypertension, diabetes, and certain cancers often develop silently, with few noticeable symptoms in the early stages. Regular check-ups and screenings can identify these issues before they become severe, allowing for early intervention and better management. For instance, mammograms and colonoscopies have been shown to reduce mortality rates from breast and colorectal cancers, respectively, by enabling early detection and treatment.

Lifestyle choices play a significant role in health outcomes. Strategic health principles emphasize the importance of nutrition, physical activity, and mental well-being. A balanced diet rich in fruits, vegetables, whole grains, lean proteins, and healthy fats provides essential nutrients that support bodily functions and reduce the risk of chronic diseases. The Mediterranean diet, for example, has been associated with lower risks of heart disease, stroke, and certain cancers. Regular physical activity, whether it's walking, swimming, or strength training, helps maintain a healthy weight, strengthens the cardiovascular system, and improves mental health. Mental well-being is another crucial aspect of health. Chronic stress, anxiety, and depression can have profound effects on physical health, contributing to conditions like heart disease and weakened immune function. Strategies to promote mental well-being include mindfulness practices, social connections, and adequate sleep. Mindfulness meditation, for example, has been shown to reduce stress and improve emotional regulation. Building and maintaining strong social relationships provide emotional support and can help buffer against stress.

Leveraging technology is another strategic element in crafting effective health principles. Digital health tools, such as wearable devices, mobile health apps, and telemedicine, have revolutionized how we monitor and manage health. Wearable devices can track physical activity, sleep patterns, and even vital signs like heart rate and blood pressure, providing real-time data that individuals can use to make informed decisions about their health. Mobile health apps offer resources for everything from tracking nutrition and exercise to managing chronic conditions like diabetes.

Telemedicine has become increasingly important,

especially in the wake of the COVID-19 pandemic. Virtual consultations allow patients to access healthcare services without the need for in-person visits, which can be particularly beneficial for those with mobility issues or who live in remote areas. According to a study published in the Journal of Medical Internet Research, telemedicine has been shown to improve access to care, enhance patient satisfaction, and reduce healthcare costs.

Community engagement and public health initiatives also play a vital role in strategic health thinking. Effective health principles often involve collaborations between individuals, healthcare providers, policymakers, and community organizations. Public health campaigns, such as anti-smoking initiatives and nutrition education programs, can raise awareness and drive behavior change on a large scale. For example, the "Truth" campaign in the United States, which targeted youth smoking, has been credited with contributing to a significant decline in smoking rates among teenagers.

Addressing social determinants of health is another key component. Factors such as socioeconomic status, education, and access to healthcare significantly influence health outcomes. Strategies that address these determinants can help reduce health disparities and promote equity. For instance, improving access to education and job opportunities can enhance economic stability and enable individuals to afford healthier lifestyles. Ensuring access to affordable healthcare services can help individuals manage their health more effectively and prevent the progression of chronic diseases.

Environmental health is an often-overlooked aspect of strategic health principles. Our surroundings, including the air we breathe, the water we drink, and the spaces we inhabit, have a profound impact on health. Efforts to reduce pollution, ensure clean water, and create safe, walkable communities contribute to overall well-being. Policies aimed at reducing emissions from industrial sources and vehicles can improve air quality and reduce respiratory conditions like asthma. Health education and literacy are foundational to effective health strategies. Empowering individuals with knowledge about their health and how to take care of it can lead to better outcomes.

Educational programs that teach skills like reading food labels, understanding prescription instructions, and recognizing symptoms of common conditions enable individuals to make informed decisions. According to the National Institutes of Health, health literacy is a critical factor in managing chronic diseases and preventing complications.

Finally, adaptability and resilience are essential qualities in strategic health thinking. The health landscape is constantly evolving, with new challenges and opportunities arising. Effective health principles must be flexible and responsive to these changes. The COVID-19 pandemic highlighted the importance of adaptability in health strategies. Swift responses, including the development and distribution of vaccines, implementation of public health measures, and adaptation of healthcare delivery systems, were crucial in managing the crisis.

In conclusion, strategic thinking in health involves a multi-faceted approach that prioritizes prevention, leverages technology, engages communities, and addresses social determinants. By focusing on these areas, we can craft effective health principles that improve outcomes and enhance the quality of life for individuals and communities. Through continuous innovation, collaboration, and education, we can build a healthier future for all.

Physical Activity: The Ultimate Longevity Enhancer

Physical activity is the ultimate longevity enhancer, and its benefits stretch far beyond weight loss or muscle gain. It plays a crucial role in maintaining overall health, preventing chronic diseases, and improving mental well-being. The science is clear: engaging in regular physical activity can extend your life, enhance its quality, and keep you feeling younger for longer. Exercise affects every part of the body, from the brain to the bones. It strengthens the heart, improving cardiovascular health and reducing the risk of heart disease. The American Heart Association recommends at least 150 minutes of moderate-intensity aerobic activity or 75 minutes of vigorous activity per week to keep the heart healthy. Activities like brisk walking, swimming, and cycling can help lower blood pressure, improve cholesterol levels, and reduce inflammation, all of which contribute to a healthier cardiovascular system.

Beyond the heart, exercise has profound effects on metabolic health. It enhances insulin sensitivity, making it easier for the body to manage blood sugar levels. This is particularly important for preventing and managing type 2 diabetes. According to the Centers for Disease Control and Prevention (CDC), regular physical activity can help prevent or delay the onset of type 2 diabetes and can help those already diagnosed to better manage their condition. Muscle contractions during exercise help cells take up glucose more efficiently, lowering blood sugar levels. Physical activity also supports bone health. Weight-bearing exercises like walking, running, and resistance training stimulate bone formation and slow down age-related bone loss. This is critical for preventing osteoporosis and fractures, particularly in older adults. The National Osteoporosis Foundation suggests that regular exercise can help maintain bone density and reduce the risk of falls and fractures. Stronger muscles from resistance training also support joint health, reducing the risk of arthritis and joint pain.

Mental health benefits from exercise are equally significant. Physical activity triggers the release of endorphins, often called "feel-good" hormones, which can alleviate symptoms of depression and anxiety. The Anxiety and Depression Association of America notes that exercise can be a powerful tool for managing mental health conditions. It reduces stress, improves mood, boosts self-esteem, and enhances cognitive function. Regular exercise has been shown to reduce the risk of developing dementia and Alzheimer's disease by promoting brain health.

Exercise also plays a crucial role in maintaining a healthy weight. By increasing energy expenditure, physical activity helps balance the calories consumed with those burned, making weight management more achievable. However, the benefits of exercise for weight management extend beyond just burning calories. It helps regulate appetite and can improve metabolic rate, making it easier to maintain a healthy weight over time.

One of the most profound impacts of regular physical activity is its ability to extend lifespan. A study published in the journal **"Circulation"** found that people who engaged in regular moderate to vigorous physical activity lived significantly longer than those who were inactive. The researchers concluded that being physically active could add years to life expectancy. Regular exercise reduces the risk of many of the leading causes of death, including heart disease, stroke, diabetes, and certain cancers. Physical activity is also essential for maintaining muscle mass and strength as we age. Sarcopenia, the age-related loss of muscle mass and function, can lead to frailty and increased risk of falls and injuries. Strength training exercises, such as lifting weights or using resistance bands, can help preserve muscle mass and improve balance and coordination. The

Mayo Clinic emphasizes the importance of incorporating strength training into a fitness routine, particularly for older adults, to maintain independence and quality of life.

Another key benefit of physical activity is its impact on sleep. Regular exercise can help improve the quality and duration of sleep, which is vital for overall health. The National Sleep

Foundation reports that people who engage in regular physical activity tend to have better sleep patterns and experience fewer sleep disturbances. Good sleep is essential for physical and mental recovery, and it plays a role in maintaining a healthy immune system.

In addition to all these benefits, physical activity can be a fun and social way to stay healthy. Group activities like sports, dance classes, or walking clubs provide opportunities for social interaction and support, which can enhance motivation and adherence to an exercise routine. Social connections are an important aspect of mental health, and combining them with physical activity can create a powerful synergy for overall well-being. It's important to find activities that you enjoy and that fit into your lifestyle. Consistency is key, and making exercise a regular part of your routine can lead to lifelong benefits. Whether it's a morning jog, a yoga class, or a game of tennis, the most important thing is to keep moving and stay active. Variety can also keep things interesting and prevent boredom, so mix up your activities to include different types of exercise.

In summary, physical activity is a cornerstone of a healthy

lifestyle. It improves cardiovascular health, supports metabolic and bone health, enhances mental well-being, aids in weight management, extends lifespan, maintains muscle mass, improves sleep, and provides social benefits. By incorporating regular exercise into your daily routine, you can enhance your longevity and enjoy a higher quality of life. The evidence is overwhelming: moving more can help you live a longer, healthier, and happier life.

Fitness Fundamentals: Preparing for Lifelong Physical Performance

Getting ready for lifelong physical performance starts with understanding the basics of fitness and making them a part of your daily routine. Fitness fundamentals lay the groundwork for a healthy and active lifestyle, whether you're aiming for peak athletic performance or simply want to stay active as you age. From building a strong foundation to developing a balanced routine, these principles can guide you on your journey to lifelong fitness.

First, let's talk about setting goals. It's essential to have clear, attainable goals to keep you motivated and focused. Goals should be specific, measurable, achievable, relevant, and time-bound (SMART). Whether you want to run a marathon, lose weight, or just improve your overall health, having a clear target can help you stay on track. For example, instead of saying "I want to get fit," you might set a goal to "run a 5k in under 30 minutes within three months."

Next, understand the importance of a balanced fitness routine. This means incorporating different types of exercises to address all aspects of fitness: cardiovascular endurance, strength, flexibility, and balance. Cardiovascular exercises like running, cycling, or swimming help improve heart and lung health. Strength training, such as lifting weights or using resistance bands, builds muscle mass and bone density. Flexibility exercises like yoga or stretching improve range of motion and prevent injuries. Balance exercises, such as tai chi or standing on one leg, help maintain stability and coordination.

A solid warm-up routine is crucial before any workout. Warming up prepares your body for physical activity by increasing blood flow to your muscles and raising your heart rate. Dynamic stretches, which involve moving parts of your body and gradually increasing reach, speed, or both, are effective. Think of movements like leg swings, arm circles, or lunges. This not only helps prevent injuries but also improves performance by enhancing muscle elasticity and flexibility. After your workout, cooling down is just as important. Cooling down helps gradually lower your heart rate and relax your muscles. Static stretches, where you hold a stretch for 15-30 seconds, can improve flexibility and reduce muscle stiffness. Focus on major muscle groups like your hamstrings, quadriceps, and shoulders. Cooling down aids in recovery and prepares your body for the next workout.

Consistency is key to lifelong fitness. It's better to engage in moderate exercise regularly than to have sporadic intense workouts. According to the American Heart Association, adults should aim for at least 150 minutes of moderate-intensity aerobic activity or 75 minutes of vigorous activity per week, along with muscle-strengthening activities on two or more days a week. Find activities you enjoy so that exercise becomes something you look forward to rather than a chore. Listening to your body is vital. Pushing yourself is important, but knowing your limits and understanding when to rest is equally crucial. Overtraining can lead to injuries and burnout. Pay attention to signs of overtraining, such as persistent fatigue, decreased performance, and mood changes. Rest and recovery are essential parts of a fitness routine. Ensure you get adequate sleep, stay hydrated, and incorporate rest days into your schedule to allow your body to repair and strengthen. Nutrition plays a significant role in fitness and performance. Fueling your body with the right nutrients helps you perform better and recover faster. A balanced diet rich in whole foods, including fruits, vegetables, lean proteins, healthy fats, and complex carbohydrates, provides the energy and nutrients needed for optimal performance. Staying hydrated is also crucial. Dehydration can impair your physical and mental performance, so make sure to drink plenty of water throughout the day, especially before, during, and after workouts. Setting realistic expectations is important for maintaining motivation and avoiding frustration. Progress in fitness takes time and patience. Celebrate small victories and milestones along the way. Remember that everyone's fitness journey is unique, and comparing yourself to others can be discouraging. Focus on your own progress and the improvements you're making, no matter how small they may seem.

Cross-training, or incorporating a variety of exercises into your routine, can prevent boredom and reduce the risk of injury. Different activities work different muscle groups and can improve overall fitness. For example, if you primarily run, adding swimming or cycling can provide a low-impact workout that still boosts cardiovascular health. Cross-training also keeps your workouts interesting and challenging, which can help maintain motivation. Tracking your progress can provide valuable insights and help keep you motivated. Use a fitness journal, mobile app, or wearable device to record your workouts, monitor your progress, and set new goals. Tracking can help you identify patterns, make adjustments to your routine, and celebrate your achievements.

Incorporating fitness into your daily life can make it easier to stick with your routine. Simple changes like taking the stairs instead of the elevator, walking or biking to work, or doing short workout sessions throughout the day can add up. Finding ways to be active in your everyday activities helps make fitness a natural and sustainable part of your lifestyle. Community support can enhance your fitness journey. Joining a fitness class, sports team, or online fitness community can provide encouragement, accountability, and social connections. Working out with others can make exercise more enjoyable and help you stay committed to your goals. Sharing your challenges and successes with a supportive community can boost your motivation and provide valuable tips and advice.

Understanding the science behind fitness can also be empowering. Learning about how different exercises affect your body, the benefits of various types of workouts, and the principles of effective training can help you make informed decisions about your fitness routine. Many reputable sources, such as the American

College of Sports Medicine and the National Institutes of Health, provide valuable information on exercise science and fitness guidelines.

Lastly, staying adaptable and open to change is essential for lifelong fitness. Your fitness needs and goals may evolve over time, and being flexible with your routine can help you stay on track. Whether you're dealing with an injury, a busy schedule, or simply looking for new challenges, being willing to adjust your approach and try new things can keep your fitness journey dynamic and rewarding. By focusing on these fitness fundamentals, you can build a strong foundation for lifelong physical performance. Regular exercise, balanced nutrition, adequate rest, and a supportive community can help you achieve your fitness goals and maintain a healthy, active lifestyle well into the future. Whether you're just starting your fitness journey or looking to enhance your current routine, these principles can guide you toward lasting success.

Movement Mastery: Preventing Injuries through Proper Mobility

Preventing injuries through proper mobility involves mastering movement patterns that keep the body safe and efficient during physical activity. Mobility isn't just about flexibility; it's about the ability of your joints and muscles to move freely and efficiently through their full range of motion. This skill is vital for athletes, fitness enthusiasts, and anyone aiming to maintain an active lifestyle.

Proper mobility starts with understanding the body's mechanics. Each joint has a specific range of motion, and muscles work in harmony to facilitate movement. When joints lack mobility, other parts of the body may overcompensate, leading to improper movement patterns and increased injury risk. For example, tight hips can cause the lower back to bear more strain during activities like running or lifting, potentially leading to back pain or injury. Dynamic warm-ups are essential for preparing the body for physical activity and enhancing mobility. Unlike static stretching, which involves holding a stretch for a prolonged period, dynamic warm-ups use movement to increase blood flow and muscle temperature.

Exercises like leg swings, arm circles, and hip openers mimic the motions you'll perform during your workout, gradually increasing the range of motion in your joints. This type of warm-up not only reduces the risk of injury but also improves performance by priming the muscles for action. Foam rolling, also known as self-myofascial release, is another effective technique for improving mobility. Foam rolling involves using a cylindrical foam roller to apply pressure to tight or sore muscles. This pressure helps break up adhesions in the muscle tissue and fascia, the connective tissue surrounding muscles. By rolling out tight spots, you can enhance blood flow, reduce muscle stiffness, and improve the flexibility and mobility of the muscles and joints. Regular foam rolling can be particularly beneficial for areas prone to tightness, such as the calves, quads, and upper back.

Strength training, when done correctly, can also enhance mobility. Building strength in the muscles surrounding a joint can improve joint stability and support proper movement patterns. For example, strengthening the muscles of the hips and glutes can improve hip mobility and reduce the risk of lower back pain. It's important to focus on exercises that promote balanced muscle development and avoid overworking any one muscle group. Compound movements, such as squats, deadlifts, and lunges, engage multiple muscle groups and joints, promoting overall mobility and functional strength. Incorporating mobility drills into your fitness routine can help maintain and improve joint function. These drills often involve controlled, repetitive movements that enhance joint range of motion and stability. For instance, shoulder circles, thoracic spine rotations, and hip hinges can keep these areas mobile and reduce the risk of injury. Practicing mobility drills regularly can help identify and address any limitations or imbalances before they lead to more serious issues.

Maintaining good posture throughout the day is crucial for mobility and injury prevention.

Poor posture, such as slouching at a desk or hunching over a smartphone, can lead to muscle imbalances and restricted joint movement. Over time, these habits can contribute to pain and injury. Practicing good posture involves being mindful of your body alignment, keeping your shoulders back, and engaging your core muscles. Ergonomic adjustments to your workspace, such as using a supportive chair and positioning your computer screen at eye level, can also help maintain proper posture. Listening to your body and recognizing the signs of overuse or strain is key to preventing injuries. Pain, discomfort, or reduced range of motion can indicate that a muscle or joint is being overworked. Rest and recovery are just as important as exercise for maintaining mobility and preventing injuries. Allowing your body time to recover between workouts can prevent overuse injuries and promote long-term joint health.

Yoga and Pilates are excellent practices for enhancing mobility and preventing injuries. Both disciplines emphasize controlled, mindful movements that improve flexibility, strength, and body awareness. Yoga poses, such as downward dog, warrior, and pigeon pose, stretch and strengthen multiple muscle groups, promoting joint mobility and stability. Pilates exercises, like the hundred, leg circles, and roll-ups, focus on core strength and controlled movement, enhancing overall body alignment and function. Hydration and nutrition also play roles in maintaining mobility and preventing injuries. Proper hydration keeps the muscles and joints lubricated, reducing stiffness and improving overall function.

Nutrients such as omega-3 fatty acids, found in fish and flaxseed, and antioxidants, found in fruits and vegetables, can reduce inflammation and support joint health. A balanced diet rich in vitamins and minerals supports muscle repair and growth, further enhancing mobility.

Sleep is another critical component of injury prevention and mobility. During sleep, the body repairs and regenerates tissues, including muscles and joints. Adequate sleep is essential for maintaining overall health and performance. Aim for 7-9 hours of quality sleep per night to support your body's recovery processes.

Education and awareness about proper movement techniques can significantly reduce the risk of injury. Working with a fitness professional, such as a personal trainer or physical therapist, can provide valuable insights into your movement patterns and identify areas for improvement. These experts can develop personalized exercise and mobility programs tailored to your needs and goals, ensuring that you move safely and effectively. Consistency in your mobility routine is key to long-term success. Incorporate mobility exercises and practices into your daily routine to maintain and improve joint function. Regular practice can lead to lasting improvements in flexibility, strength, and overall movement quality, reducing the risk of injury and enhancing your ability to perform daily activities and athletic pursuits.

In summary, mastering movement and preventing injuries through proper mobility involves a combination of dynamic warm-ups, foam rolling, strength training, mobility drills, good posture, mindful movement practices like yoga and Pilates, proper hydration and nutrition, adequate sleep, and education. By integrating these elements into your fitness routine, you can enhance your mobility, prevent injuries, and maintain an active and healthy lifestyle for years to come.

Next-Level Nutrition: The Science Behind Our Food Choices

What we choose to eat shapes our health, energy levels, and overall well-being. Next-level nutrition takes us beyond basic dietary guidelines and delves into the science behind our food choices. Understanding the biochemical impact of different nutrients, the role of gut health, and the importance of personalized nutrition can revolutionize how we approach our diets. At the core of next-level nutrition is the recognition that food is more than just fuel. It's a complex mix of nutrients, enzymes, and chemicals that interact with our bodies in complex ways. Carbohydrates, proteins, and fats are the macronutrients that provide energy, but they do so in different ways. Carbohydrates break down into glucose, the body's primary energy source.

However, not all carbs are created equal. Simple sugars cause rapid spikes in blood sugar, leading to crashes, while complex carbs, like those in whole grains, provide sustained energy and support digestive health. Proteins, made up of amino acids, are the building blocks of muscles, tissues, and organs. They play a crucial role in repair and growth. The body requires twenty different amino acids, nine of which are essential and must be obtained through diet. Animal products are complete protein sources, providing all essential amino acids, whereas most plant-based proteins are incomplete and need to be combined to ensure adequate intake.

Fats, often misunderstood, are essential for health. They support cell structure, hormone production, and nutrient absorption. Unsaturated fats, found in nuts, seeds, avocados, and fish, are beneficial, whereas trans fats and excessive saturated fats can increase the risk of chronic diseases. Omega-3 and omega-6 fatty acids, types of unsaturated fats, are particularly important for brain health and reducing inflammation. Micronutrients, including vitamins and minerals, are equally vital. Vitamins like A, C, D, E, and the B-complex support various bodily functions, from immune defense to energy production. Minerals such as calcium, magnesium, and potassium are critical for bone health, nerve function, and muscle contraction. Deficiencies in these nutrients can lead to severe health issues, making it important to consume a varied diet rich in fruits, vegetables, lean proteins, and whole grains.

The gut microbiome has emerged as a critical player in next-level nutrition. This community of trillions of bacteria, viruses, and fungi in our digestive tract affects everything from digestion to immunity to mental health. A balanced microbiome supports nutrient absorption and helps prevent pathogens from taking hold. Fiber-rich foods like fruits, vegetables, legumes, and whole grains feed beneficial bacteria, promoting a healthy gut environment. Probiotics, found in fermented foods like yogurt, kefir, and sauerkraut, can also boost the population of good bacteria. Personalized nutrition recognizes that individual responses to food vary. Factors like genetics, age, gender, activity level, and health status influence dietary needs. For instance, some people have genetic variations that affect how they metabolize caffeine or certain fats. Others might have intolerances or sensitivities to foods like gluten or lactose. Personalized nutrition uses tools like genetic testing, blood biomarkers, and microbiome analysis to tailor dietary recommendations to individual needs. This approach can optimize health outcomes and reduce the risk of chronic diseases.

The timing of eating, or meal timing, is another aspect of next-level nutrition. Intermittent fasting, which involves alternating periods of eating and fasting, has gained popularity for its potential benefits on metabolism, weight management, and even longevity. Studies suggest that intermittent fasting can improve insulin sensitivity, support cellular repair processes, and reduce inflammation. However, it's important to approach fasting carefully, especially for individuals with certain health conditions. Hydration is a fundamental yet often overlooked aspect of nutrition. Water is essential for nearly every bodily function, from regulating temperature to transporting nutrients. Dehydration can impair physical and cognitive performance, cause headaches, and affect mood. While the common recommendation is to drink eight glasses of water a day, individual needs can vary based on factors like activity level, climate, and overall health. It's important to listen to your body and drink when thirsty, but also to be mindful of signs of dehydration.

The quality of food is as important as its quantity. Organic foods, free from synthetic pesticides and fertilizers, are often perceived as healthier, though the evidence is mixed. What's clear is that minimally processed foods, free from additives and preservatives, are generally better for health. Whole foods like fresh fruits, vegetables, lean meats, and whole grains are nutrient-dense and support overall well-being. Processed foods, high in added sugars, unhealthy fats, and sodium, contribute to obesity, heart disease, and other chronic conditions.

Sustainability is becoming an essential consideration in next-level nutrition. The environmental impact of food production, including greenhouse gas emissions, water use, and land use, influences the health of the planet and its inhabitants. Plant-based diets, which emphasize vegetables, fruits, legumes, nuts, and seeds, are generally more sustainable than diets heavy in animal products. Reducing meat consumption, choosing locally sourced and seasonal foods, and minimizing food waste can contribute to a healthier planet.

Behavioral aspects of eating also play a significant role. Mindful eating, which involves paying attention to hunger and fullness cues, savoring food, and eating without distractions, can improve digestion, reduce overeating, and enhance the overall eating experience. Emotional eating, where food is used to cope with stress or emotions, can lead to unhealthy eating patterns and weight gain. Developing a healthy relationship with food involves recognizing emotional triggers and finding alternative ways to cope with stress. Food allergies and intolerances are important considerations in next-level nutrition. Food allergies, involving the immune system, can cause severe reactions and require complete avoidance of the allergen. Common allergens include peanuts, tree nuts, shellfish, and dairy. Intolerances, like lactose intolerance, involve the digestive system and cause discomfort but are generally less severe. Identifying and managing food allergies and intolerances is crucial for health and well-being.

Understanding the impact of food on mental health is another frontier of next-level nutrition. Certain nutrients, like omega-3 fatty acids, B vitamins, and antioxidants, support brain health and can influence mood and cognitive function. Diets high in processed foods and low in nutrients have been linked to increased risk of depression and anxiety. Conversely, diets rich in whole foods, lean proteins, and healthy fats support mental well-being.

Next-level nutrition is about making informed choices based on science, individual needs, and a holistic understanding of health. It involves not just what we eat, but how, when, and why we eat. By embracing the principles of next-level nutrition, we can enhance our health, performance, and quality of life.

Practical Nutrition: Developing a Personalized Eating Plan

Creating a personalized eating plan isn't just about following a set diet; it's about understanding your unique nutritional needs and preferences. This approach ensures that your eating habits are sustainable and enjoyable while supporting your health and fitness goals. Here's how you can develop a practical nutrition plan tailored to you.

Start by identifying your goals. Are you aiming to lose weight, gain muscle, improve your energy levels, or manage a health condition? Your goals will guide your dietary choices. For example, if weight loss is your objective, you'll need to create a calorie deficit by consuming fewer calories than you burn. On the other hand, if you want to build muscle, you'll require a calorie surplus with an emphasis on protein intake.

Next, assess your current eating habits. Keep a food diary for a week, noting everything you eat and drink. This will help you identify patterns and areas for improvement. Are you skipping meals, overeating at certain times, or consuming too much sugar and processed food? Understanding your baseline is crucial for making informed changes.

Macronutrients: carbohydrates, proteins, and fats – are the foundation of your diet. Each plays a specific role in your body. Carbohydrates are your body's primary energy source, proteins are essential for muscle repair and growth, and fats support cell function and hormone production. Balancing these macronutrients according to your goals is key. For instance, athletes might need more protein for muscle recovery, while someone managing diabetes might need to focus on low glycemic index carbs to maintain stable blood sugar levels.

Personal preferences and lifestyle also play significant roles in developing a personalized eating plan. Consider your likes and dislikes, dietary restrictions, and cultural or ethical beliefs. If you're vegetarian or vegan, ensure you're getting enough protein from plant-based sources like beans, lentils, and tofu. If you have food allergies or intolerances, identify safe and nutritious alternatives. Customizing your plan to fit your lifestyle increases the likelihood of sticking with it long-term.

Meal timing and frequency can influence your energy levels and metabolism. Some people thrive on three square meals a day, while others prefer smaller, more frequent meals. Intermittent fasting, which involves alternating periods of eating and fasting, has gained popularity for its potential health benefits, including improved insulin sensitivity and weight management. Find an eating pattern that fits your schedule and feels natural for you.

Hydration is an often-overlooked aspect of nutrition

but is vital for overall health. Water supports digestion, nutrient absorption, and temperature regulation. Aim to drink at least eight glasses of water a day, more if you're active or live in a hot climate. Infusing water with fruits or herbs can make it more appealing if you find plain water boring.

Portion control is essential, especially if your goal is weight management. Understanding serving sizes and listening to your body's hunger and fullness cues can prevent overeating. Using smaller plates, eating slowly, and avoiding distractions during meals can help you better recognize when you're satisfied. Incorporate a variety of foods to ensure you're getting a broad spectrum of nutrients. Fruits and vegetables provide vitamins, minerals, and antioxidants. Whole grains like brown rice, quinoa, and oats offer fiber and energy. Lean proteins from sources like chicken, fish, beans, and nuts support muscle maintenance and repair. Healthy fats from avocados, olive oil, and fatty fish support brain health and inflammation control. Eating a rainbow of foods ensures you're not missing out on essential nutrients.

Planning and prepping meals in advance can save time and help you stick to your eating plan. Batch cooking, using leftovers creatively, and keeping healthy snacks on hand can prevent the temptation to opt for convenience foods that may not align with your goals. For example, cooking a large batch of quinoa or roasting a tray of vegetables can provide the basis for multiple meals throughout the week.

Monitoring and adjusting your plan is crucial for long-term success. Regularly check in with yourself to see how you're feeling physically and emotionally. Are you meeting your goals? Are there any challenges or areas where you're struggling? It's normal to make adjustments as you go. If you're not seeing the results you want or if your needs change, don't be afraid to tweak your plan.

Working with a nutrition professional can provide personalized guidance and support. Dietitians and nutritionists can help you create a plan tailored to your specific needs and goals. They can also provide accountability and help you navigate any challenges or barriers you encounter. This professional support can be especially valuable if you have specific health conditions or complex dietary needs.

Education is a powerful tool in developing a personalized eating plan. Learning about nutrition, reading food labels, and understanding how different foods affect your body can empower you to make informed choices. Knowledge enables you to navigate social situations, dining out, and food marketing more effectively, ensuring you stay on track with your plan. Sustainability should always be a consideration. A diet that's too restrictive or doesn't consider your preferences and lifestyle is unlikely to be maintained in the long run. The goal is to create an eating plan that supports your health and well-being while being enjoyable and realistic. Flexibility, allowing for occasional treats and indulgences, is important for maintaining a healthy relationship with food.

Mindful eating practices can enhance your nutrition plan. Paying attention to what and how you eat, savoring each bite, and recognizing hunger and fullness cues can improve digestion and satisfaction. Avoiding emotional eating and addressing stress through other means can also support your nutritional goals.

Your social environment and support system can impact your

eating habits. Surround yourself with people who support your goals and create an environment that makes healthy choices easier. This might involve cooking with family, joining a health-focused community group, or seeking support from friends who share similar goals.

Developing a personalized eating plan involves understanding your goals, assessing your current habits, balancing macronutrients, considering personal preferences and lifestyle, and staying hydrated. It includes mindful eating, portion control, and planning ahead. Regular monitoring, education, professional support, and sustainability are crucial for long-term success. By taking these steps, you can create a nutrition plan that's tailored to your unique needs and

supports your overall health and
well-being.

Sleep Optimization: Embracing Rest for Cognitive Health

Sleep is a fundamental pillar of cognitive health, yet it's often neglected in our fast-paced world. Optimizing sleep isn't just about getting enough hours in bed; it's about enhancing the quality of that sleep to improve brain function, mood, and overall health.

First, understanding the different stages of sleep is crucial. Sleep isn't a uniform state but a complex process with several stages, each serving a specific purpose. Non-rapid eye movement (NREM) sleep includes three stages: light sleep (stages 1 and 2) and deep sleep (stage 3). Rapid eye movement (REM) sleep is when most dreaming occurs. Deep sleep is essential for physical recovery and immune function, while REM sleep is critical for cognitive functions like memory consolidation and mood regulation. Ensuring you progress through these stages multiple times each night is key to sleep optimization.

Creating a sleep-friendly environment can significantly impact sleep quality. Your bedroom should be cool, dark, and quiet. These conditions promote the body's natural sleep rhythms. Use blackout curtains to block out light, invest in a comfortable mattress and pillows, and consider white noise machines or earplugs if noise is an issue. Keeping electronic devices out of the bedroom is also important, as the blue light emitted by screens can interfere with the production of melatonin, the hormone that regulates sleep.

Consistency is another vital aspect of sleep optimization. Going to bed and waking up at the same time every day helps regulate your internal clock, making it easier to fall asleep and wake up naturally. Even on weekends, try to maintain your sleep schedule. This consistency reinforces your body's sleep-wake cycle and can improve the quality of your sleep over time.

Diet and exercise also play roles in sleep quality. Consuming caffeine and nicotine close to bedtime can disrupt sleep, as both are stimulants. Similarly, while alcohol might help you fall asleep initially, it can interfere with the deeper stages of sleep, leading to a less restful night. On the other hand, regular physical activity can promote better sleep. However, try not to exercise too close to bedtime, as this can be stimulating and make it harder to fall asleep.

Stress and mental health are closely linked to sleep quality. High stress levels can make it difficult to fall asleep or cause fragmented sleep. Techniques such as mindfulness, meditation, and deep-breathing exercises can help manage stress and improve sleep. Establishing a pre-sleep routine that includes relaxing activities like reading, taking a warm bath, or practicing yoga can signal to your body that it's time to wind down and prepare for sleep.

Exposure to natural light during the day, particularly in the morning, can help regulate your sleep-wake cycle. Light influences the production of melatonin, so getting plenty of daylight helps keep your circadian rhythms in sync.

Conversely, reducing exposure to artificial light in the evening can help signal to your body that it's time to prepare for sleep. Dimming the lights and avoiding screens in the hour before bed can make a big difference.

Nutritional choices also impact sleep. Foods rich in magnesium, such as leafy greens, nuts, and seeds, can promote relaxation and improve sleep quality. Tryptophan, found in turkey, chicken, and bananas, can increase the production of serotonin and melatonin, aiding sleep. Avoid large meals and heavy, rich foods within a few hours of bedtime, as these can cause discomfort and disrupt sleep.

Technology can both help and hinder sleep. While screens and blue light can interfere with melatonin production, several apps and devices are designed to promote better sleep. Wearable devices can track sleep patterns, helping you identify issues and make adjustments. Sleep apps can offer guided meditations, white noise, and other tools to help you relax and fall asleep. Smart lighting systems can gradually dim the lights in the evening, mimicking the natural sunset and signaling to your body that it's time to wind down.

Mental health conditions such as anxiety and depression often go hand-in-hand with sleep disturbances. Addressing these conditions can significantly improve sleep quality. Cognitive behavioral therapy for insomnia (CBT-I) is an effective treatment for chronic sleep issues, helping to change negative thought patterns and behaviors around sleep. Seeking support from a mental health professional can be a crucial step in improving both sleep and overall well-being.

Circadian rhythms, the body's internal clock, regulate the sleep-wake cycle. Disruptions to these rhythms, such as from shift work or travel across time zones, can wreak havoc on sleep. Strategies to realign your circadian rhythms include exposing yourself to natural light during the day, using light therapy, and gradually adjusting your sleep schedule before traveling. Understanding and respecting your body's natural sleep-wake cycle can lead to more restorative sleep.

Sleep disorders like sleep apnea, restless leg syndrome, and chronic insomnia require medical attention. Sleep apnea, characterized by repeated interruptions in breathing during sleep, can lead to severe health issues if untreated. Treatment options include lifestyle changes, CPAP machines, and in some cases, surgery. Restless leg syndrome, causing uncomfortable sensations and an urge to move the legs, can also disrupt sleep. Medications and lifestyle changes can help manage this condition. Chronic insomnia, characterized by difficulty falling or staying asleep, often requires a multifaceted approach, including behavioral therapy and medication.

Monitoring and adjusting your sleep habits are essential for long-term success. Keeping a sleep diary can help you track patterns and identify triggers for poor sleep. Note when you go to bed, when you wake up, and the quality of your sleep. This information can help you make informed adjustments to your routine and environment.

Incorporating relaxation techniques into your daily routine can improve sleep quality. Progressive muscle relaxation, guided imagery, and aromatherapy are all effective ways to calm the mind and prepare for sleep. Creating a relaxing bedtime ritual that you look forward to can make a significant difference in your ability to fall asleep and stay asleep.

Finally, recognizing the value of sleep is crucial. In a culture that often prioritizes productivity over rest, it's important to understand that sleep is not a luxury but a necessity. Quality sleep supports cognitive function, emotional regulation, physical health, and overall well-being. Prioritizing sleep is an investment in your health that pays off in every aspect of your life.

By optimizing your sleep, you can enhance your cognitive health, improve your mood, and increase your overall quality of life.

Emotional Wellness: The Critical Role of Mental Health in Longevity

Emotional wellness is a key aspect of overall health, directly impacting longevity. Mental health isn't just about avoiding mental illness; it's about fostering a state of well-being where individuals can cope with the normal stresses of life, work productively, and contribute to their communities. Achieving emotional wellness involves managing stress, building resilience, maintaining positive relationships, and finding purpose.

Stress management is crucial for emotional wellness. Chronic stress can lead to numerous health problems, including heart disease, hypertension, diabetes, and mental health disorders like anxiety and depression. Learning how to manage stress effectively can significantly improve quality of life and longevity. Techniques such as mindfulness meditation, deep breathing exercises, and progressive muscle relaxation can help reduce stress. Mindfulness involves staying present in the moment and observing thoughts and feelings without judgment. This practice has been shown to reduce stress, enhance emotional regulation, and improve overall well-being.

Building resilience is another essential component of emotional wellness. Resilience is the ability to bounce back from adversity, trauma, or significant sources of stress. It involves behaviors, thoughts, and actions that anyone can learn and develop. Key strategies for building resilience include maintaining a positive view of yourself, accepting change as a part of life, and keeping things in perspective.

Establishing goals and taking decisive actions rather than detaching from problems and wishing they would go away can also strengthen resilience.

Positive relationships provide support, create opportunities for joy, and reduce feelings of loneliness and isolation. Strong social connections have been linked to lower risks of many significant health problems, including high blood pressure, unhealthy body mass index (BMI), and a reduced risk of death. Cultivating relationships involves effective communication, empathy, and regular interaction. Participating in community activities, volunteering, and joining groups with shared interests can help build and maintain these connections.

Finding purpose and meaning in life contributes significantly to emotional wellness and longevity. Having a sense of purpose has been associated with numerous health benefits, including a longer life span, reduced risk of disease, and improved mental health. Purpose can come from work, volunteering, learning new skills, or nurturing relationships. It involves setting goals that align with your values and making progress toward them.

Mental health conditions like depression and anxiety can significantly affect emotional wellness and longevity. Depression is a common but serious mood disorder that affects how you feel, think, and handle daily activities. Symptoms can include persistent sadness, loss of interest in activities, and difficulty concentrating. Anxiety disorders involve excessive fear or worry that interferes with daily activities. Both conditions can be treated with therapy, medication, and lifestyle changes. Seeking help from a mental health professional is crucial if you're experiencing symptoms of these disorders.

Self-care practices play a vital role in maintaining emotional wellness. Regular physical activity, a healthy diet, sufficient sleep, and avoiding harmful behaviors like smoking or excessive alcohol consumption are fundamental. Exercise, in particular, has been shown to have significant benefits for mental health, including reducing anxiety, depression, and negative mood, and improving self-esteem and cognitive function. Physical activity increases the production of endorphins, chemicals in the brain that act as natural painkillers and mood elevators. Healthy eating also supports emotional wellness. Diets rich in fruits, vegetables, whole grains, and lean proteins can improve mood and energy levels. Certain nutrients, such as omega-3 fatty acids, found in fish, and antioxidants, found in fruits and vegetables, have been linked to lower rates of depression. Avoiding processed foods, sugary snacks, and excessive caffeine can also help maintain stable energy levels and mood.

Adequate sleep is essential for emotional wellness. Sleep affects mood, cognitive function, and physical health. Chronic sleep deprivation can lead to a range of health issues, including impaired memory, weakened immunity, and increased risk of mental health disorders. Establishing a regular sleep routine, creating a restful environment, and avoiding screens before bed can improve sleep quality.

Emotional intelligence, the ability to understand and manage your own emotions and recognize and influence the emotions of others, is crucial for emotional wellness. High emotional intelligence can help you navigate social complexities, lead and motivate others, and excel in your personal and professional life. Developing emotional intelligence involves improving self-awareness, self-regulation, social skills, empathy, and motivation.

Seeking support when needed is an important aspect of emotional wellness. Whether it's talking to a trusted friend, family member, or mental health professional, having someone to confide in can help manage stress and emotional challenges. Professional help can provide strategies to cope with stress, manage mental health conditions, and improve emotional well-being.

Technology can be both a help and a hindrance to emotional wellness. While social media and digital communication can enhance connections, they can also lead to feelings of inadequacy and isolation. It's essential to use technology mindfully, setting boundaries to ensure it enhances rather than detracts from your emotional wellness. Tools like mental health apps can provide resources for mindfulness, stress management, and tracking mood and habits.

Cultural and societal factors also influence emotional wellness. Social norms, values, and expectations can impact how individuals perceive and manage their emotions. Promoting a culture that values mental health, reduces stigma, and encourages seeking help can improve emotional wellness on a broader scale. Policies that support mental health, such as access to care, mental health education, and workplace wellness programs, are crucial.

Emotional wellness is a dynamic and multifaceted aspect of health that plays a critical role in longevity. By managing stress, building resilience, nurturing relationships, finding purpose, practicing self-care, developing emotional intelligence, seeking support, and being mindful of cultural influences, individuals can enhance their emotional well-being and overall quality of life. Recognizing the importance of mental health and taking proactive steps to support it can lead to a longer, healthier, and more fulfilling life.